THE GOOD ENERGY COOKBOOK

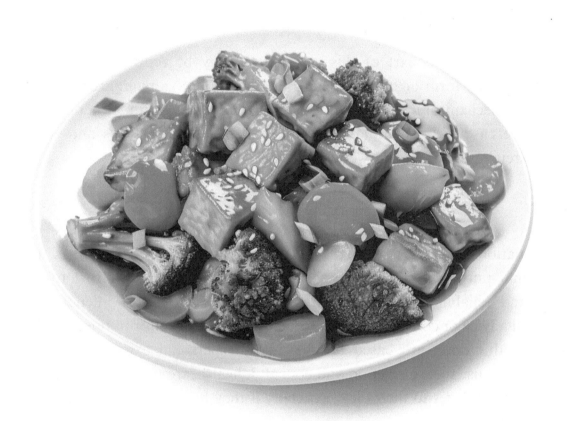

Over 80 Recipes Inspired by Dr. Casey Means' Teachings to Help You Lose Weight, Improve Overall Health, and Boost Your Metabolic Function

Jacqueline L. Payne

Disclaimer

The information provided in **"THE GOOD ENERGY COOKBOOK"** is for general informational purposes only. While the author has made every effort to ensure the accuracy and reliability of the information presented, it is not intended to replace professional advice or consultation. The recipes, nutritional information, and health tips provided in this book are based on the author's personal experience and research. Readers should use their discretion and consult a healthcare professional before making any significant changes to their diet, especially if they have specific health conditions or dietary restrictions.

The author and publisher disclaim any liability for any damages or adverse effects arising from the use of the information contained in this book. The reader assumes full responsibility for their actions.

Letter To The Reader

Greetings, Reader

Have you ever caught yourself blaming your metabolism for your inability to lose weight, regardless of your efforts? My metabolism is too sluggish") or making light of the metabolism of others ("She's fortunate to have a quick metabolism"). Why is there a difference in her ability or incapacity to lose weight when she can eat anything she wants and not gain weight? Then you are not by yourself. In actuality, I spent a considerable amount of time beside you.

I had categorized myself as belonging to the group of people who had a slow metabolism. I reasoned that I would need to put in a lot more effort than most if I wanted to lose weight and keep it off. But eventually I saw that this wasn't the case. I didn't have to put in more effort. I have to work more efficiently.

Your metabolism is dynamic, which means it is always changing rather than fixed. This means that your everyday choices have a significant impact on how your metabolism functions, which is a huge benefit for weight loss and overall health.

You hold the power since your metabolism is mostly influenced by your hormones, stress levels, activity level, and body composition—how much muscle and fat you have. By making varied everyday decisions, you have the power to alter your hormone balance, decrease stress, boost exercise levels, and alter your body composition.

It takes time to transform your metabolism into a productive calorie-burning machine, but the effort is well worth it. I hope you'll come along.

I'm wishing you the best possible health and well-being.

Jacqueline L. Payne

Introduction

It's normal in today's world to mistreat your body. The current standard of processed foods, high-stress lifestyles, and little leisure time can lead to health issues. This poisonous combination eventually harms the body and leads to mistaken blame.

When struggling to lose weight, it's common to blame your metabolism. For example, "I just can't lose weight no matter what I do." I've got a slow metabolism." That might be true right now, but was it always this way? And must it stay that way? Both of these enquiries have the same answer: no.

Contrary to popular belief, metabolism is not fixed and can be altered. Your metabolism is not stagnant. It is continually altering and evolving based on the information it receives from your body. Your metabolism is affected by what you eat, how much you move, how you deal with stress, and your overall mood.

Poor eating habits, lack of sleep, insufficient exercise, exposure to toxins, and a fast-paced lifestyle have all contributed to your current metabolic state. These decisions have altered your biochemistry by altering hormonal signalling in your body.

This was a gradual transformation that occurred over time. You may not have seen it until you paused for a moment and looked in the mirror. You suddenly find yourself overweight, weary, and cranky. You can hardly get through lunch without wanting to fall asleep at your desk at work. You cannot go on like this. Something needs to change.

The difficulty is, you may not know where to begin. Making healthy decisions can restore your metabolism to its original level, allowing you to achieve your optimum weight and feel more energetic and clear.

Eating complete, nutrient-dense foods, exercising frequently, getting enough sleep, and reducing stress not only feels good, but also helps regulate hormones and restore balance. Your body wants to perform properly and healthily; it just has a difficult time doing so when it lacks the necessary tools.

It may take some time to restore your metabolism to its optimal state, just as it did to reach your current level. The good news is that when you treat your body well, you'll start to notice changes in a matter of days that will encourage you to continue on your current course. You may notice that your pants fit more comfortably, you are less bloated, you are able to rise from bed without hitting the snooze button multiple times, or your skin appears brighter and softer. These are all signs that your hormones are resetting and you are on the path to a healthy, happy metabolism. When you begin to treat your body with kindness, it will reciprocate by being kind to you.

Who Is Casey Means

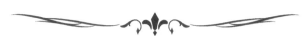

Dr. Casey Means is a prominent figure in the field of metabolic health and wellness. She is a Stanford-trained physician who specializes in the intersection of metabolism, health, and technology. Dr. Means is the co-founder and Chief Medical Officer of Levels, a health technology company that focuses on metabolic fitness through continuous glucose monitoring. Her work aims to empower individuals to understand and optimize their metabolic health to improve overall well-being.

In addition to her role at Levels, Dr. Means is known for her contributions to the medical and health community through her writing and research. She has been a vocal advocate for preventive healthcare, emphasizing the importance of lifestyle and dietary choices in managing chronic diseases.

Dr. Means is also an author and recently published the book "Good Energy: The Surprising Connection Between Metabolism and Limitless Health," where she explores the profound impact of metabolism on various aspects of health and provides insights into achieving optimal energy and vitality through metabolic awareness.

Her work has been featured in various publications, and she is a sought-after speaker on topics related to health, wellness, and technology.

Overview Of Casey Means Teachings

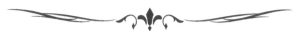

Dr. Casey Means' Good Energy is a groundbreaking exploration of the vital connection between metabolism and overall health. The book challenges conventional wisdom by asserting that many common health issues, from fatigue and brain fog to chronic diseases, can be traced back to metabolic imbalances.

Central to Means' argument is the concept of "good energy". This refers to the optimal energy production within our cells, which is essential for physical and mental well-being. She introduces a framework called the "Cellular Energy Equation" to explain how various factors, including diet, exercise, sleep, stress, and environment, impact our metabolic health.

Good Energy provides a comprehensive guide to optimizing metabolism and achieving limitless health. It offers practical, evidence-based strategies for improving energy levels, boosting cognitive function, and preventing chronic diseases. By emphasizing the importance of metabolic balance, Means empowers readers to take control of their health and well-being. Essentially, the book posits that by understanding and optimizing our metabolism, we can unlock our full potential for vibrant health and vitality.

How This Cookbook Can Help You

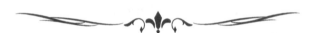

The Good Energy Cookbook offers readers a practical application of Dr. Casey Means' groundbreaking concepts from Good Energy. By translating her metabolic principles into delicious and nourishing recipes, the cookbook empowers readers to:

- Achieve Weight Loss Goals: The recipes are designed to support

- weight loss by focusing on whole foods, balanced macronutrients, and portion control.
- Boost Metabolism: The cookbook incorporates ingredients known to support a healthy metabolism, helping readers burn calories efficiently and maintain energy levels.
- Improve Overall Health: By providing recipes rich in essential nutrients, the cookbook contributes to overall well-being, including improved digestion, stronger immunity, and better skin health.
- Enhance Energy Levels: The focus on metabolic health ensures that the recipes provide sustained energy throughout the day, reducing fatigue and brain fog.
- Simplify Healthy Eating: The cookbook offers a variety of flavorful and satisfying meals, making it easier for readers to adopt a healthy eating lifestyle without feeling deprived.

In essence, The Good Energy Cookbook is more than just a collection of recipes; it's a roadmap to transforming your relationship with food and achieving optimal health through the power of good energy.

Chapter 1

Understanding Metabolism

The term "metabolism" is often used. You have likely heard statements such as, "I am unable to lose weight due to my slow metabolism," or "You are extremely fortunate to have such a fast metabolism." You have the freedom to consume any food you desire without accumulating excess weight. Although these statements provide a fundamental grasp of how your metabolism regulates your weight, it's only the beginning. Your metabolism is far more than that. The chemical processes within your body are what keep you alive, not just one "thing" as some may believe.

What Is Metabolism?

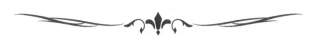

Metabolism refers to the chemical reactions that transform food into energy for various bodily functions such as movement, thinking, growth, and sleep. Every second, thousands of metabolic events occur in your body simultaneously. Metabolic activity fall into two categories: catabolic and anabolic.

Types of Metabolism

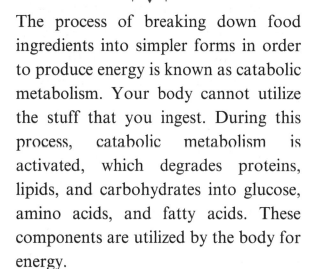

The process of breaking down food ingredients into simpler forms in order to produce energy is known as catabolic metabolism. Your body cannot utilize the stuff that you ingest. During this process, catabolic metabolism is activated, which degrades proteins, lipids, and carbohydrates into glucose, amino acids, and fatty acids. These components are utilized by the body for energy.

Anabolic metabolism takes over when catabolic metabolism has completed its task. The leftover materials from catabolic metabolism are used by anabolic metabolism to create new bodily tissues and cells. Additionally, some elements might be saved as energy for later use.

FACTS: All chemical reactions are propelled by energy released during catabolic processes. Adenosine triphosphate, or ATP, is the energy that is stored there. The amount of ATP that the human body can hold at any given moment is just approximately 9 ounces (250 grams), yet it is constantly recycled and used again.

Hormones regulate both kinds of metabolism. Similar to metabolism, the hormones that influence weight and metabolism are classified as either catabolic or anabolic. For a healthy metabolism, you require both anabolic and catabolic hormones. The secret is to keep these hormones in the right balance with a healthy diet and way of living.

The Major Hormones

Hormones influence your body's reactions. The goal of your body's hormonal system, also known as the endocrine system, is to preserve homeostasis, or perfect equilibrium. Endocrine glands produce and release more of a hormone in response to a decrease in blood levels of that hormone. Endocrine glands produce less hormones in response to increases in blood hormone levels. In a healthy body, this system functions flawlessly. When a body experiences malnourishment, excessive stress, and exposure to toxins in the environment, the delicate hormonal balance can be disrupted.

Insulin

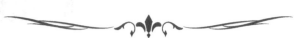

One of the most talked-about hormones and a key component of your metabolism is insulin. Insulin primarily lowers blood sugar by binding to and transporting glucose molecules from the bloodstream to your cells. Your blood sugar rises shortly after eating a meal, particularly one that contains a lot of refined carbs, since glucose is released into the bloodstream. The organ that lies just below your stomach, the pancreas, releases insulin into your bloodstream in reaction to this spike in blood sugar.

One of three functions of insulin is to transport glucose to the cells so they can be used as fuel right away; it also transports glucose to the liver where it is transformed into glycogen and stored for use as fuel when the body doesn't have access to glucose from meals; and finally, it aids in the conversion of glucose into fatty acids, which are subsequently stored as fat in your fat cells. That's part of the purpose of this program—your body uses the energy from these fatty acids when there isn't any glucose.

The Way Insulin Deviates

The simple explanation for why your body stops responding to insulin properly is overexposure. When you consume large amounts of refined carbohydrates, such as pasta, bread, desserts, and sugar, your blood sugar levels become chronically elevated. In an attempt to counteract this, your pancreas releases excessive amounts of insulin, which quickly removes glucose from your bloodstream, causing your blood sugar to drop and leaving you feeling hungry and wanting more of these carbs.

Important Notice: According to estimates from the Centers for Disease Control and Prevention, 29.1 million Americans today have diabetes, and nearly 30% of those individuals are unaware that they have the disease. It's critical to manage your hormone levels if you suspect insulin resistance in order to prevent diabetes from developing.

Although your body may initially be capable of managing this cycle, the cells eventually cease to respond effectively to the excess insulin. Right now, your insulin levels are elevated in addition to your blood sugar. Insulin resistance is what this is, and it's a big risk factor for metabolic syndrome and type 2 diabetes.

Signs of Insulin Imbalance

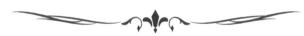

Hormonal imbalance is only one

example of how well your body can alert you to problems. Typical indicators of an insulin imbalance include:

- Obesity in the abdomen
- Acne
- Hazy vision
- Dark skin patches on the folds of the body (neck, groin, and armpits)
- Depression
- Inability to fall or keep asleep
- Feeling tired
- Not being able to reduce weight
- Increased urination and thirst

Thyroid

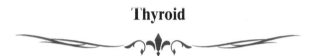

Your thyroid hormones are the next important metabolic factor. Located somewhat above the collarbone and below the actual or potential Adam's apple, your thyroid gland is a butterfly-shaped organ. Iodine is a mineral that your thyroid uses to create two distinct thyroid hormones: T3 (triiodothyronine) and T4 (thyroxine). Following their release into the bloodstream, these hormones regulate metabolism, or the process by which calories are turned into energy. Your body's metabolism is dependent on these thyroid hormones for every single cell. About 80% of T4 and 20% of T3 are produced by a thyroid gland that is healthy and functioning. The hormonal potency of T3 is four times that of T4.

The pituitary gland, a little organ located near the base of the brain, regulates the thyroid gland. Thyroid-stimulating hormone (TSH) is produced by the pituitary gland and instructs the thyroid to release hormones in response to decreased blood levels.

How Unbalanced Thyroid Hormones Occur

Prolonged stress, poor nutrition, pollutants in the environment, severe diets, some drugs, and inflammatory disease processes can all affect your thyroid. In the event that one or more of these are present, your thyroid may react by slowing down or accelerating. You may become hypothyroid (having too few thyroid hormones) or hyperthyroid (having too many thyroid hormones) as a result.

Importance Notice: An imbalance in the thyroid can be quite problematic. Make an appointment with your healthcare provider to have your thyroid levels evaluated if you suspect either an underactive or hyperactive thyroid.

Signs of Thyroid Imbalance

The following are some typical indicators that your thyroid hormone levels are low:

- Fog in the brain
- Rough skin and hair
- Bewilderment Constipation
- Depression
- Having trouble swallowing
- Desiccated skin
- Exhaustion
- Heavy times
- Intolerance for the cold
- Hair loss cramping in the muscles
- Slow-moving heartbeat
- Gaining weight

Having too much thyroid hormone can manifest as a number of symptoms:

- Diarrhea
- wooziness
- Exhaustion Hyperactivity
- Elevated heart rate
- Increased perspiration
- Lack of sleep
- Intolerance
- Anxiety/nervousness
- Loss of weight

Fight-or-Flight Hormones

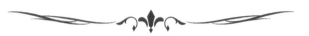

In situations where you are in immediate danger, the fight-or-flight response is meant to save your life. Consider it this way: Your forefathers had to hunt and gather food in the past. Every now and again they would encounter something potentially fatal, like a tiger. The body releases adrenaline, cortisol, and norepinephrine in the single second it takes to decide whether to run away from the tiger or fight it.

Insulin production is halted by norepinephrine. This is done to keep glucose in the blood so that, in an emergency, you have access to a rapid supply of energy.

In order to reduce blood supply to the stomach and intestines, epinephrine relaxes the muscles in these regions and halts digestion. This is done to increase blood flow to the extremities, which will improve your ability to run or fight. Cortisol tells your body to stop releasing adrenaline and norepinephrine and return to normal when the acute stress has passed.

Importance Notice: Human cortisol secretion typically occurs in a daily or diurnal cycle. Naturally, cortisol levels rise as soon as you wake up and then gradually fall over the day. This normal cycle may be reversed in a person with a cortisol imbalance, leading to higher cortisol levels at night and lower levels first thing in the morning.

Although this hormone reaction is very helpful when you need to act quickly in difficult situations, the continuous stress of modern life has made it problematic. A lot of people have elevated cortisol levels because they are always in a fight-or-flight mode. Cortisol is a catabolic hormone, meaning that it breaks down things, which is why this is an issue. Stretch marks and osteoporosis can result from elevated cortisol levels, which also damage down muscle, bone, and epidermis. Cortisol furthermore instructs your body to retain fat in the belly. This explains why having too much abdominal fat is linked to high stress levels.

How Stress Hormones Go Out of Control

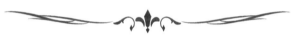

The adrenal glands, which are the glands that sit on top of your kidneys and create these hormones, become overstimulated by prolonged stress, which can be caused by poor food, excessive work, and insufficient relaxation. An increased sensitivity to stress results from the chronic activation of this stress response. This feedback loop gets stronger with time, to the point where even small threats will result in a significant stress reaction.

Signs of Cortisol Imbalance

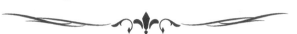

Typical indicators of an imbalance in cortisol include:

- Ambiguity
- Abdominal fat
- Depression
- Diarrhea
- Skin that bruises easily
- Weary
- Blood pressure that is high or low
- Lack of sleep
- Insulin sensitivity
- Erratic times
- Appetite decline
- Yearning for salt
- Gained or lost weight

The Steroid Hormones

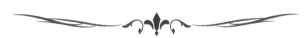

Estrogen, progesterone, testosterone, and dehydroepiandrosterone (DHEA) are the steroid hormones, which are occasionally referred to as the sex hormones. Both men and women contain both hormones, although in varying amounts. While estrogen and progesterone are typically associated with women, testosterone and DHEA are typically linked with men. To keep your metabolism functioning efficiently, you must keep your body in the proper balance.

Estrogen and Progesterone

Numerous functions are played by estrogen, particularly in the body of a woman. Development, digestion, heart health, electrolyte balance, memory, and bone density are all impacted by estrogen. Although a woman's body has many other forms of estrogen, estradiol, estrone, and estriol are the three primary forms. It is more common in younger women to have estradiol. It keeps a woman's physique slim and helps decrease blood pressure and insulin. Moreover, it controls energy levels, mood, and hunger. Estrone replaces estradiol as the primary estrogen hormone when you get older. Your body receives an estrogen signal to store fat. One byproduct of estradiol metabolism is estriol. Estriol exhibits weaker estrogenic action in comparison to estradiol and estrone.

When testosterone and estrogen levels are balanced in men, estrogen has minimal impact on metabolism. However, excessive estrogen levels can result in fat storage and a loss of lean muscular mass.

How Estrogen Gets Out of Control

Many dismiss estrogen-related issues as an inevitable byproduct of aging. Although it's true that hormone levels change with age, you have the power to alter your destiny by your decisions. Numerous substances can mimic the effects of estrogen. Your body reacts to these compounds by increasing fat storage, lowering libido, and inducing depression and anxiety, among other things. Your body interprets these chemicals as growing estrogen levels. So what is the source of these chemicals? They are the artificial chemicals in your kitchen cleaner, the scent in your perfume, and the preservatives in your food. You literally can't get away from them.

Signs of Estrogen Imbalance

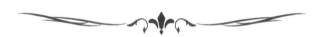

Among the typical indicators of an estrogen excess in women are:

- Uncertainty
- Bloating and belly fat
- Fog in the brain
- Cravings for carbohydrates
- Diminished desire for things
- Depression
- lightheadedness
- Tiredness and dry skin
- Hair thinning
- PMDD/PMS

Among the symptoms of an estrogen excess in men are:

- Diminished desire for things

- Reduced tone of the muscles
- Depression
- Impotence
- surplus breast tissue
- A rise in body fat
- Low number of sperm

Testosterone and DHEA

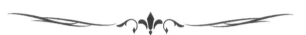

By definition, androgen hormones, which include testosterone and DHEA, are anabolic hormones. Instead of destroying, they usually increase muscle. In both sexes, testosterone aids in the growth of lean muscular mass, strength, libido, and vitality. The testes supply the majority of a man's body's DHEA and testosterone. The adrenal glands produce DHEA and testosterone in a female's body.

How Androgens Get Out of Control.

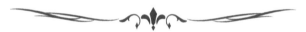

Your body naturally begins to produce less DHEA and testosterone as you get older. This creates a Catch-22 situation. Reduced drive to exercise and greater fat storage are the results of androgen hormone decline. Your body turns testosterone into estrogen when there is an increase in fat storage, which lowers levels even further. When you combine becoming older with a diet high in refined carbohydrates and low in nutrients, your body will produce less

DHEA and testosterone.

Signs of Androgen Hormone Imbalance

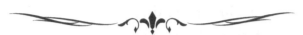

Typical indications of an imbalance in androgen hormones include:

- Aggression Due to Acne
- Uncertainty
- Abdominal fat
- Modifications to the makeup of the body
- Diminished desire for things
- Depression
- Impotence
- Weary
- hair thinning
- lowered voice
- Decreased density of bones

Ghrelin and Leptin

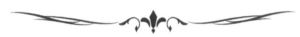

The hunger hormones are leptin and ghrelin. The small intestine and stomach release ghrelin. It lets your body know when food is ready. Ghrelin levels rise in people with healthy, active metabolisms after periods of fasting and fall as they begin to feel full.

Ghrelin is reversed by leptin. Your body uses leptin to tell you when to stop eating. It lets the brain know that there is enough fat stored in the body. The issue is that, even with larger blood levels of leptin, your body doesn't react to it efficiently if you're overweight or your metabolism is out of whack. You thus never feel satisfied after eating a large meal.

How Leptin and Ghrelin Get Out of Control

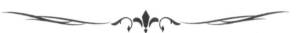

What then triggers the imbalance in these hormones? You guessed it: the way you live. The main issue here is an imbalance in leptin, although oddly enough, low leptin levels aren't usually the cause of the issue. In actuality, studies have shown that blood levels of leptin are typically greater in those with higher body fat percentages. The issue is that your brain's leptin-responsive receptors become inactive when you consistently overeat, consume foods heavy in unhealthy carbs or trans fats, don't get enough sleep, and lead a life full of ongoing stress. This condition is known as leptin resistance, and it coexists alongside insulin resistance.

Signs of Leptin Resistance

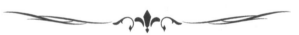

Among the typical indicators of leptin resistance are:

- Ongoing hunger
- Depression
- Diabetes
- Elevated blood pressure

- Inflammatory response
- Being overweight

How Did You Get Here?

You're probably wondering how you got here and, more importantly, what you can do about it if any of the symptoms and hormone problems sound like you. To successfully execute the lifestyle modifications that will reset your metabolism, you must first grasp the "how." Many individuals want to place the responsibility straight away on heredity, but that's only one piece of the puzzle—and sometimes a little one. Although genetics do influence your body's functioning, experts believe that this influence is only 10–30%, depending on the ailment. The saying "Your genes load the gun, and your environment/choices pull the trigger" may not be familiar to you. The key takeaway is that, even if your genetic makeup predisposes you to something, your lifestyle choices greatly influence which genes express and which ones do not.

Poor Diet

There are certain foods on the market nowadays that are a complete nightmare for a healthy metabolism. For what reason is that the case?

because processed, commercially generated food isn't even recognized as food by your body. Artificial chemicals, preservatives, high sugar content, and genetically modified organisms (GMOs) are all present in these lab-made foods. Your biochemistry can be harmed more by foods that have undergone greater processing. In addition, these processed foods lack the nutrients your body requires to survive, making them unrecognizable as food. Some producers attempt to circumvent this by adding vitamins and minerals to processed foods, but your body can only absorb a portion of these artificial substances.

Importance Notice: Natural vitamin B1 was found to be 1.38 times more effectively absorbed than a single synthetic vitamin B1 molecule in an animal investigation. The efficiency of absorption increased 1.92 times for vitamin B2 and 3.94 times for vitamin B3.

An excessive, or yo-yo, diet history is associated with poor diet. Severe diets, such as extremely low-calorie plans, prolonged juicing, or cleanse-style diets deficient in nutrients, throw off your hormonal equilibrium by telling your metabolism to shut down in the event that this "famine" lasts longer than expected and food becomes scarce. Catabolic diets cause your body to break down your muscles in order to produce energy. You have to put in more effort to lose weight since your body is less able to burn calories at rest when you have less lean muscle mass.

Not Enough Exercise

While it's true that as you get older, your body produces less hormones overall, new study suggests that you may be able to slow down this process more than you may believe. Exercise, in combination to a healthy diet, contributes to increased lean muscle mass and natural hormone balance. Three times as many calories are burned for every pound of muscle as there are for every pound of fat. This implies that your metabolism gets more effective as you increase your amount of lean muscle and decrease your body fat.

The Question?
Which kind of exercise is best for me?

Include physical activity of all kinds in your weekly schedule. The greatest effect for hormone balance comes from combining cardiovascular activity, like jogging, with strength-training exercises, like lifting weights, and stress-relieving exercises, like yoga or tai chi.

Conversely, inactivity causes hormone

levels to drop, body fat to grow, and metabolism to become disrupted.

Overwhelming Stress—and Insufficient Stress Reduction

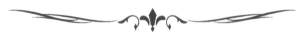

Prolonged stress, even mild amounts of it, can seriously mess with your hormones. This hormonal disturbance brought on by stress is linked to weight gain and a slowed metabolism. Although you can't totally avoid stress, it's still vital to manage your stress levels on a daily basis.

Too Little Sleep

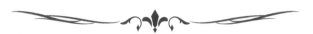

Lack of sleep is a common side effect of excessive stress. You start to give up sleep in order to finish your work when your stress levels increase. Perhaps you're rising too early to engage in a workout, or perhaps you stay up too late to finish that crucial task. Perhaps insomnia or a lack of quality sleep has been brought on by the overanalyzing that comes with stress. For whatever reason, one of the main contributors to hormone imbalance associated with stress is insufficient sleep.

Your body makes less leptin and more ghrelin when you're sleep deprived. Your body will therefore continuously advise you to eat without alerting you when it's time to quit. Not getting enough sleep causes your metabolism to slow down as well, which reduces how effectively you use the calories you eat.

Environmental Toxicity

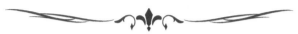

An important factor contributing to disturbance of hormones and metabolism that is not discussed nearly enough is environmental toxicity. Nearly 100,000 synthetic compounds are currently registered for usage in commerce, and thousands more are added every year. Processed foods, cosmetics, skincare products, household cleaning supplies, plastics, and other items include these artificial compounds. The issue is that a significant portion of these artificial chemicals have never even undergone safety testing, and those that have been shown to be endocrine disruptors. This implies that exposure to these artificial substances can upset your hormonal balance, even at extremely low concentrations. Numerous health problems, such as weight gain, autoimmune illnesses like asthma and Hashimoto's thyroiditis, allergic reactions, and cancer, might result from this.

Chapter 2

Breakfast Recipes

Apple-Cinnamon Quinoa Porridge

Ingredients
Serves 2

- 1/2 cup of quinoa
- 1 small Granny Smith apple, cored and minced
- 3/4 cup of water
- 1 tsp finely ground cinnamon
- 1/8 teaspoon of salt

Steps
- Use cold water to rinse the quinoa until the water turns clear. Use cheesecloth or a fine strainer to drain the quinoa.
- All ingredients should be combined in a medium saucepan over medium-high heat. After bringing the mixture to a boil, turn down the heat.
- After the water is absorbed and the quinoa is tender, cook it covered for 15 to 20 minutes.
- Take off the heat and leave it covered for five minutes. Using a

fork, fluff the mixture, then divide it equally between two bowls. Warm up and serve.

Peach Pear Smoothie

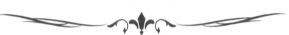

Ingredients
Serves 2

- 1/3 of a cup of frozen peaches
- 1/3 cup frozen pears
- 1/4 tsp finely powdered cinnamon
- 1 cup of coconut water
- 1 tablespoon freshly squeezed lemon juice
- 1 cup of fresh spinach.

Steps
- Blend all of the ingredients until they are smooth.

Overnight Oats

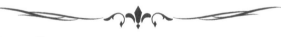

Ingredients
Serves 2

- 1/2 cup of steel-cut oats

- 1/2 cup of strawberries
- 1/2 cup of blueberries.
- 1/4 tsp finely powdered cinnamon
- 1/8 tsp ground nutmeg
- 2 glasses of water.

Steps

- In a large bowl, combine the oats, berries, cinnamon, and nutmeg. Add water to the mixture and whisk until well blended.
- Place the mixture in the fridge with a cover on for the entire night. Take the mixture out of the fridge in the morning and reheat it in a medium-sized saucepan over low heat for 20 minutes, stirring now and then.
- Warm up and serve.

Spirulina Power Smoothie

Ingredients
Serves 2

- 1 cup of water
- 1 small, sliced cucumber
- 1 tiny green apple, cut into slices and cored
- 1/2 cup frozen berry mixture
- 2 teaspoons spirulina
- 1 teaspoon of granulated stevia (optional).

Steps

- In a blender, combine all ingredients and process until smooth.

Blueberry French Toast

Ingredients
Serves 2

- 1 cup of blueberries, frozen
- 1 tsp lemon juice
- 1/4 teaspoon powdered stevia
- 1/8 teaspoon of salt.
- 2 big egg whites
- 2 tsp of essence from vanilla
- 1/2 tsp finely ground cinnamon
- 2 pieces of bread with sprouts

Steps

- Place the blueberries in a small skillet and cook over medium heat for about five minutes, or until the blueberries begin to bubble and pop. Mix in salt, stevia, and lemon juice until the fruit mixture has the right consistency. Put aside.
- In small basin, whisk egg whites, cinnamon, and vanilla. Make careful to coat both sides of each sprouted bread slice by soaking it in the mixture.
- After transferring the bread to a medium skillet, fry it over medium heat, rotating it once to brown it on both sides.
- Place the French toast on a platter and drizzle half of the berry mixture over each slice. Warm up and serve.

Mango Pineapple Smoothie

Ingredients
Serves 2

- ½ cup fresh mango, cubed
- ½ cup fresh pineapple, cubed
- 3 tablespoons freshly squeezed lemon juice
- 1 cup ice cubes.
- 1 cup of water

Steps
- In a blender, combine all ingredients and process until smooth.

Chicken Apple Sausage with Scrambled Egg Whites

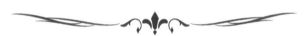

Ingredients
Serves 2

- 1 tsp water
- 1 (3-ounce) chicken apple sausage link (no sugar added) cut into small pieces.
- 1 cup of finely chopped spinach
- 4 big egg whites
- 1/4 tsp salt of garlic
- 1/4 of a teaspoon of black pepper, ground

Steps
- Fill a small skillet with water and

heat it to medium. After adding the sausage, throw it in the hot skillet and turn it occasionally until it browns. After the sausage has browned, add the spinach to the pan and cook for three minutes, or until it wilts.
- Whisk the egg whites, garlic, salt, and pepper in a another medium bowl. Over the sausage mixture, pour the egg mixture, and scramble for 3–4 minutes, or until done.
- Present warm.

Blueberry-Lemon Quinoa Porridge

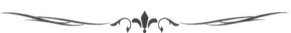

Ingredients
Serves 2

- 1/2 cup of quinoa
- 1 cup of water
- 1/8 teaspoon of salt
- Zest of a big lemon
- 1/2 cup blueberries
- 1 tsp ground flax seed
- 1 tsp finely chopped stevia

Steps
- Till the water runs clear, rinse the quinoa under cold water. Use cheesecloth or a fine-mesh sieve to drain the quinoa.
- Place quinoa and water in a medium saucepan and heat over high heat until they reach a simmer. When mixture begins to boil, add

- salt, lower heat to low, cover, and simmer for about 20 minutes, or until all water has been absorbed.
- Take the saucepan off the burner and use a fork to fluff the quinoa. Stir in stevia, flaxseed, blueberries, and zest from the lemon. Warm up and serve.

Metabolism-Boosting Smoothie

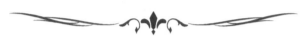

Ingredients
Serves 2

- 1 cup of coconut water
- ½ cup of green iced tea without sugar
- ¼ cup of florete broccoli
- 1 cup of strawberries, frozen
- 1/4 cup washed and drained canned cannellini beans
- 1/2 tsp finely ground stevia
- 1½ teaspoon of cinnamon powder
- 1/8 teaspoon of grated ginger

Steps
- Blend all of the ingredients until smooth.

Breakfast Stuffed Sweet Potatoes

Ingredients
Serves 2

- 1 medium sweet potato, cut in half

- horizontally
- 2 tsp water
- 1/2 tsp finely chopped garlic
- 1/4 cup finely diced yellow onion
- 1 cup of finely chopped spinach
- 4 big egg whites
- 1/2 tsp salt
- 1/4 teaspoon of black pepper, ground
- 1/2 teaspoon powdered onion

Steps
- Turn the oven on to 400°F. On a baking pan, place the sweet potato cut-side down. Bake the sweet potato for 25 minutes, or until it is tender.
- After the sweet potato is cooked, bring a medium skillet of water to a simmer. Add the onion and garlic, and simmer for about five minutes, or until tender. Cook the spinach for three minutes, or until it has wilted.
- Whisk the egg whites with the onion powder, salt, and pepper in a medium-sized bowl. After adding the egg mixture to the spinach mixture, scramble the eggs until they are fully cooked. Take off the heat.
- Using a fork, mash the sweet potato flesh inside the skin. Place half of the egg mixture over each half of the sweet potato. Warm up and serve.

Amaranth Breakfast Porridge

Ingredients
Serves 2

- 1 cup of water
- 1/2 cup of amaranth
- 1½ teaspoon of cinnamon powder
- 1/4 teaspoon of allspice powder
- 1 tsp finely chopped stevia
- 1/2 cup of raw blueberries

Steps

- Place the amaranth and water in a small saucepan and raise it to a boil over high heat. Once the majority of the water has been absorbed, reduce heat to low and simmer for 20 minutes. Avoid overcooking.
- Stir in stevia, cinnamon, and allspice. Spoon into two serving bowls; garnish with the fresh blueberries. Serve right away.

Vegetable Frittata

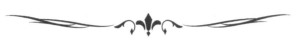

Ingredients
Serves 2

- 1 teaspoon of water.
- Chop ½ medium zucchini
- ½ chopped, peeled, medium yellow onion
- 1 cup of spinach
- 6 big egg whites
- 1 tablespoon of freshly chopped parsley
-
- 1/4 tsp salt
-
- 1/8 teaspoon of black pepper, ground

Steps

- Set oven temperature to 350°F. Heat a medium skillet over medium-high heat and add water to the pan while the oven preheats. Simmer the onion and zucchini for five minutes, or until they are tender.
- Cook the spinach for three minutes, or until it wilts.
- Turn off the heat on the vegetable combination.
- Beat the egg whites, parsley, salt, and pepper in a medium-sized basin.
- Evenly distribute the veggie mixture on the bottom of an 8" by 8" pan. Cover with egg mixture.
- Bake for 20 minutes, or until the eggs are thoroughly cooked.

Oatmeal Smoothie

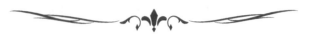

Ingredients
Serves 2

- 1 cup steel-cut oatmeal
- 1 cup of ice

- 1 cup of mixed frozen berries
- 1 tsp finely shredded fresh ginger
- 1 teaspoon of granulated stevia (optional).

Steps

- Blend all the ingredients in a blender until smooth. Serve right away.

Open-Faced Breakfast Sandwich

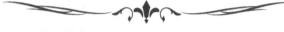

Ingredients
Serves 2

- 4 slices of turkey bacon.
- 2 pieces of bread with sprouts
- 4 big egg whites.
- 1/2 tsp salt
- 1/4 teaspoon of black pepper, ground
- 1 tsp water

Steps

- A medium skillet should be heated to medium-high heat. In a heated skillet, add the turkey bacon. After 3 minutes of cooking, turn over. Cook for a further three minutes, or until well cooked and browned. Put aside.
- Toast the sprouted grain bread while the bacon cooks.
- Whisk the eggs, salt, and pepper in a small bowl. With the water heated to a medium temperature, add the

egg mixture to the skillet. Take around three minutes to scramble the eggs until they are fully done.
- Place two pieces of turkey bacon on each slice of toast, then cover each with half of the egg mixture. Serve right away.

Cinnamon Pumpkin Smoothie

Ingredients
Serves 2

- 1 cup of pumpkin purée.
- 1 cup of water
- 1/4 teaspoon of cinnamon powder
- 1/4 tsp vanilla essence
- 1/48 tsp ground ginger
- 1 teaspoon of spirulina

Steps

- In a blender, combine all ingredients and process until smooth. Serve right away.

Turkey Fruit Salad

Ingredients
Serves 2

- 5 ounces of chopped, sugar-free smoked turkey breast
- 1 cup of cantaloupe, cubed
- 1 cup of honeydew cubes
- 1/2 cup of celery, cut
- 1 tsp freshly squeezed lemon juice

- 1 tablespoon finely chopped scallions (only the green portion)

Steps
- In a bowl, mix the turkey breast, cantaloupe, honeydew, and celery. Mix in some lemon juice. Add chopped scallions on the top.
- Put in the fridge for half an hour. Present cold.

Strawberry Pineapple Smoothie

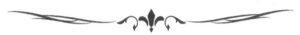

Ingredients
Serves 2

- 1/2 cup of fresh, hulled strawberries
- 1/2 cup of fresh pineapple, cubed
- 2 tsp freshly squeezed lime juice
- 1 cup ice cubes.
- 1 cup of water
- 1/8 teaspoon of finely chopped, fresh ginger

Steps
- In a blender, combine all ingredients and process until smooth.

Quinoa Breakfast Bowl

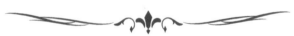

Ingredients
Serves 2

- 1/2 cup of well-rinsed and drained quinoa

- 1 cup of water
- 2 Tbsp chicken broth
- 2 tsp finely chopped white onion
- 6-large egg whites
- 1/2 cup cherry tomatoes cut in half
- Salmon smoked in four ounces

Steps
- In a small saucepan, combine the quinoa and water; come to a boil over high heat. After the water reaches a boil, lower the heat to a simmer, cover, and let the quinoa cook for 20 minutes, or until it becomes tender. Take off the heat and give it five minutes.
- Heat the broth in a medium skillet over medium-high heat. Add the onion and simmer for about 5 minutes, or until transparent. Scramble the egg whites until they are fully cooked.
- Add the fish and tomatoes, then fully cook. Place the quinoa in the skillet and mix thoroughly. Serve right away.

Egg White Breakfast Burrito

Ingredients
Serves 1

- 1 tablespoon water
- 1 tablespoon finely chopped red pepper
- 1 tablespoon finely chopped green

- pepper
- 1 tablespoon finely chopped yellow pepper
- 1 tablespoon finely chopped red onion
- 4 big egg whites
- 1 cooked slice of chopped turkey bacon
- 1/2 tsp salt
- 1/4 teaspoon of black pepper, ground
- 1 tortilla with sprouted grains

Steps

- In a medium skillet, heat the water over medium-high heat. Add the onion and peppers, and simmer for about 5 minutes, or until tender.
- In a larger bowl, whisk together the egg whites and add them to the onion and pepper combination. Get scurrying. Add salt, pepper, and turkey bacon to the eggs as they begin to cook. After 3–4 minutes, or until the eggs are set, keep cooking.
- Take off the heat, place on a tortilla, and wrap the tortilla like a burrito. Serve right away.

Egg White "Muffins"

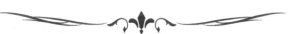

Ingredients
Serves 6

- 2 cups of egg whites, or roughly 24 of them

- 2 cups of baby spinach
- 1 small red bell pepper, chopped and seeded
- ½ cup finely minced white mushrooms.
- 1/2 tsp salt
- 1/4 teaspoon of black pepper, ground
- Set oven temperature to 350°F.

Steps

- Cupcake liners are used to line each well of a twelve-cup muffin tray.
- In a medium bowl, whisk together all the ingredients and evenly spoon the egg mixture into each muffin tray. Bake the egg for 20 to 25 minutes, or until set.

Chapter 3

Lunch Recipes

Open-Faced Turkey Sandwich

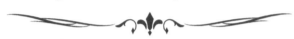

Ingredients
Serves 2

- 2 pieces of bread with sprouts
- 2 tsp yellow mustard
- 1 medium-sized fresh fig
- 1/2 cup baby spinach
- 6 ounces of roasted, sliced turkey breast

Steps

- Toast the bread with sprouts. Apply one teaspoon of yellow mustard on each slice.
- Slice the fig lengthwise, then use a spoon to remove the insides.
- Place half of the fig on a slice of toast. Add cup baby spinach and 3 ounces of turkey breast on the top of each slice.

Taco Bowls

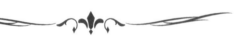

Ingredients
Serves 2

- 1 cup of brown rice
- 1 1/2 cups of water
- 1/2 pound lean ground beef.
- 1 cup washed and drained canned black beans
- Taco seasoning, 2 tablespoons
- 1½ cups of shredded lettuce.
- 1/4 cup salsa (without added sugar)

Steps

- In a medium saucepan, combine the rice and water; bring to a boil. After the mixture reaches a boiling point, turn down the heat to low, cover, and simmer for 20 minutes, or until the water has been completely absorbed.
- Heat a medium skillet over medium heat while the rice cooks.
- Add the ground beef to the hot skillet and cook until it turns no longer pink. When the meat is done, add the beans and stir until they reheat. Mix in taco seasoning after adding it.
- After dividing the rice between two bowls equally, place half of the beef and bean mixture on top of each .

- bowl.
- Add / cup shredded lettuce and / cup salsa to the top of each bowl

Massaged Kale and Apple Salad

Ingredients
Serves 2

- 4 cups of kale
- 1 medium lemon's juice
- 1/4 tsp sea salt
- ½ chopped medium cucumber
- 1 medium Granny Smith apple, cored, diced
- 2 tsp finely chopped red onion
- 1/2 cup washed and drained canned chickpeas
- ½ a tsp balsamic vinegar
- 1/4 tsp freshly ground black pepper

Steps
- Combine sea salt, lemon juice, and kale in a big bowl. For about three minutes, massage the ingredients together until the kale begins to wilt.
- Toss to mix in the cucumber, apple, onion, chickpeas, vinegar, and pepper.
- Split equally between two bowls for serving. Serve right away.

Hearty Lentil Soup

Ingredients
Serves 4

- 2 tablespoons plus 2 cups of water.
- 1 small yellow onion, peeled and sliced
- 2 celery stalks, chopped
- 2 medium carrots, cut into cubes and peel
- 2 minced garlic cloves
- 4 cups of broth made with vegetables
- 1 cup of washed and drained dry lentils
- 1/2 tsp salt
- 1/2 teaspoon of black pepper, ground
- 1 tsp of Italian spice
- ½ cup finely chopped spinach

Steps
- Heat two teaspoons of water in a large stockpot over medium heat.
- After it's hot, add the onion, celery, and carrots and cook for about five minutes, or until tender. Add the garlic and simmer for about 3 minutes, or until fragrant.
- Stir together lentils, broth, and the remaining water. Reduce the heat to low and let it simmer.
- After simmering, incorporate Italian seasoning, salt, and pepper. Simmer the lentils for 30 to 45 minutes, or until they are tender.
- After the lentils are tender, use an immersion blender to puree half of

the soup, or use a standard blender. Add the spinach after combining the puréed and nonpuréed soups. Warm up and serve.

Brown Rice Stir-Fry

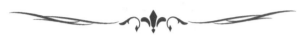

Ingredients
Serves 2

- 1 cup brown rice.
- 1 1/2 cups water.
- 2 tablespoons coconut aminos.
- 1 small yellow onion, peeled and chopped
- 1/2 medium red bell pepper, seeded and chopped
- 1/2 medium green bell pepper, seeded and chopped.
- 1 medium, diced zucchini.
- 6 ounces boneless, skinless chicken breast, cut into 1" pieces.
- 1 teaspoon of spicy sauce.
- 1/4 teaspoon salt
- 1/8 teaspoon ground black pepper.
- 1/2 cup pea shoots.

Steps
- Cook rice and water in a small pot over high heat.
- After bringing to a boil, lower the heat to a simmer and cover. Simmer for 20 minutes to soften the rice.
- Place the coconut aminos in a wok or big skillet over medium heat.
- Add the onion and simmer for

about 5 minutes, or until transparent. Cook until the peppers are tender, approximately 5 minutes. Cook zucchini till tender, but still somewhat crunchy.
- Add the chicken and simmer for about 10 minutes, or until no longer pink. Stir in the spicy sauce, salt, and pepper.
- Turn off the heat. Spoon half of the stir-fry mixture over each of the two bowls of rice that you have equally divided. Arrange cup pea shoots on top of each bowl. Serve warm.

Savory Bacon and Chive Oatmeal

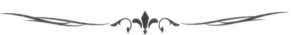

Ingredients
Serves 2

- 4 slices of sugar-free turkey bacon
- 1 1/2 cups chicken stock.
- 1/2 cup water.
- 1/2 cup steel-cut oats.
- 2 tablespoons of chopped fresh chives, plus one tablespoon for garnish.
- 1/4 teaspoon salt
- 1/4 teaspoon ground black pepper.

Steps
- Turn the heat up to medium-high in a medium skillet. Place bacon in skillet and cook for 4-5 minutes on each side, or until browned and crispy. Take the bacon from the fire and set it aside.

- Bring the stock and water mixture to a gentle boil over high heat in a medium saucepan. Add steel-cut oats and decrease heat to low.
- Simmer for twenty to twenty-five minutes, stirring from time to time, or until liquid is absorbed.
- While the oats cook, roughly cut the bacon. Add the bacon bits, two tablespoons of chives, salt, and pepper after the liquid has been absorbed. Sprinkle with the remaining 1 tablespoon chives. Serve warm.

Lemon Shrimp with Brown Rice Linguini

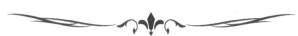

Ingredients
Serves 4

- 6 glasses of water
- 8 oz brown rice linguine
- 1/2 cup of chicken stock
- ½ cup vinegar made from white wine
- Juice of 1 big lemon
- 1/4 tsp salt
- 1/4 teaspoon of black pepper, ground
- 1/8 teaspoon of lemon pepper
- 1 pound of uncooked medium shrimp, peeled and deveined
- 1/8 cup of parsley, chopped

Steps
- Fill a big stockpot with water and

- heat it to a boil over high heat. Cook the brown rice linguini for about 7 minutes, or until it's al dente.
- After draining, set away.
- Mix the broth, vinegar, and lemon juice in a big skillet over a medium heat. Bring to a boil, cover, and cook for approximately ten minutes, or until the sauce has thickened and reduced by half.
- Stir in the lemon pepper, black pepper, and salt after adding them. Cook for an additional minute.
- Add the shrimp and simmer for about 3 minutes, or until pink. Cover the brown rice linguini with the shrimp and sauce combination. Add parsley on top. Serve right away.

Sprouted Tuna Wrap

Ingredients
Serves 2

- 1 (5-ounce) canned tuna packed in water
- Peel and chop 2 big hard-boiled eggs, removing the yolks and chopping the whites.
- 2 tsp yellow mustard
- 1 tablespoon finely chopped white onion
- 1/2 tsp seasoned salt
- 1/4 teaspoon of black pepper, ground

- 2 tortillas with sprouted grains
- 1/2 cup pea shoots

Steps

- Tuna, chopped egg whites, mustard, onion, seasoned salt, and pepper should all be mixed in a medium-sized bowl.
- Top each tortilla with an equal amount of tuna mixture and / cup pea shoots. Tortillas should be rolled out and toothpicked. Serve right away.

Three-Bean Chili

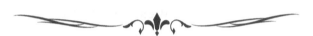

Ingredients
Serves 8

- 4 cups vegetable broth
- 1 small yellow onion, peeled and diced
- 1 large red pepper, seeded and diced
- 1 small jalapeño pepper, seeded and diced
- 1 (15-ounce) can black beans, drained and rinsed
- 1 (15-ounce) can red kidney beans, drained and rinsed
- 1 (15-ounce) can white cannellini beans, drained and rinsed
- 1 cup dried lentils, rinsed and drained
- 1 (15-ounce) can crushed tomatoes
- 1 (15-ounce) can fire-roasted diced tomatoes

- 1 tablespoon chili powder
- 1 teaspoon ground cumin
- ½ teaspoon garlic powder
- ½ teaspoon onion powder
- ½ teaspoon salt
- ¼ teaspoon ground black pepper
- ¼ cup chopped fresh cilantro

Steps

- In a slow cooker, combine all the ingredients (except the cilantro) and cook on low for 8–10 hours or on high for 4–6 hours.
- If preferred, top heated servings with cilantro.

Mustard-Roasted Salmon

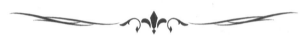

Ingredients
Serves 2

- 2 (6-ounce) salmon fillets.
- 3 Tbsp spicy mustard
- 1 tsp white vinegar
- 1/2 tsp salt
- 1/2 teaspoon of black pepper, ground
- 1/4 cup finely chopped shallots

Steps

- Turn the oven on to 400°F. Place the salmon fillets on top of a baking sheet that has been lined with parchment paper.
- Mix the mustard, vinegar, shallots, salt, and pepper in a small bowl.

- Over each filler, equally distribute the mustard mixture in a thin layer.
- Salmon should be baked for 15 to 20 minutes, or until it flakes easily. Serve right away.

Sweet Potato and Black Bean Burrito

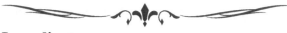

Ingredients
Serves 4

- 2 medium-sized sweet potatoes, chopped and skinned
- 1½ teaspoon of cinnamon powder
- 1/4 tsp fine-grain sea salt
- 1 (15-ounce) can black beans, drained and rinsed.
- 1½ teaspoon of cumin powder
- 1/4 tsp powdered garlic
- 1/4 teaspoon powdered onion
- 1/8 teaspoon of cayenne
- 4 tortillas with sprouted grains
- 1/2 tsp spicy sauce (without additional sugar)

Steps

- Turn the oven on to 400°F. Put parchment paper on one baking sheet and set it aside.
- Sweet potatoes should be combined with coarse sea salt and cinnamon in a medium-sized bowl. Arrange potatoes evenly on the baking pan. Bake for 20 to 25 minutes, rotating once, or until the sweet potatoes are tender and crisp.

- Preheat a small skillet to medium heat while the potatoes are cooking. Add cumin, cayenne, onion powder, and garlic powder to the skillet with the beans. Cook for about 6 minutes, or until beans are heated and seasonings are blended. Take off the heat.
- After the potatoes are cooked, transfer them to a medium-sized bowl along with the beans. Evenly distribute the contents among the tortillas, and if preferred, drizzle with hot sauce. Using a toothpick, fasten the wrapped burrito. Serve right away.

Lemon Chicken Breast

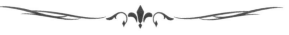

Ingredients
Serves 2

- 1/2 tsp salt
- 1/2 teaspoon of black pepper, ground
- 1½ teaspoon of peppercorns
- 1/4 teaspoon of paprika, smoked
- 1/4 teaspoon of dehydrated parsley
- 2 (4 ounce) boneless, skinless chicken breasts
- 2 tablespoons of chicken broth.
- 1 big lemon
- 2 tsp finely chopped, recent parsley

Steps

- In a plastic bag the size of a gallon,

- combine salt, black pepper, lemon pepper, paprika, and parsley. Shake thoroughly to combine. To coat the chicken breasts with the spice mixture, place them in the bag and shake.
- In a big skillet over medium heat, preheat the broth. When the chicken is no longer pink, add the breasts and cook for 5 minutes on each side.
- Squeeze lemon juice over each breast of the chicken just before it's done cooking.
- Stem fresh parsley on top and remove from heat. Serve right away.

Sardine Salad

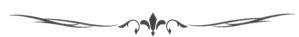

Ingredients
Serves 2

- 4 cups of mixed greens
- 1 medium lemon's juice
- 3 tablespoons of balsamic vinegar (no sugar added)
- 1/2 tsp salt
- 1/4 teaspoon of black pepper, ground
- 1/4 cup finely diced beets
- ½ cup finely chopped tomatoes
- 1/2 cup of celery, chopped
- 1 (4.3-ounce) can of sardines packed in water.

Steps
- Mix the mixed greens, vinegar, lemon juice, salt, and pepper in a big basin. Toss to thoroughly combine. Add tomatoes, cucumbers, and beetroot on top, then mix once more.
- Sardines should be chopped and topped with salad. Serve right away

Turkey Meatloaf

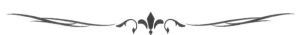

Ingredients
Serves 4

- 2 tablespoons of chicken broth.
- 1 cup of finely chopped white onion
- 3 cloves of minced garlic
- 1 lb of turkey, ground
- 1/4 cup of steel-cut oatmeal
- 2 big egg whites
- 1/4 cup sugar-free ketchup, divided
- 2 tsp of coconut aminos
- 1/2 tsp salt
- 1/2 teaspoon of black pepper, ground

Steps
- Turn the oven on to 350°F.
- In a medium skillet, heat the broth over medium heat. Add the onion and garlic, and simmer for about 5 minutes, or until transparent. Take off the heat and place aside.
- Turkey, oats, egg whites, / cup ketchup, coconut aminos, salt, and

- pepper should all be combined in a big dish. Add the mixture of onions and garlic. Blend thoroughly.
- Transfer the turkey mixture to a loaf pan and pour the remaining ½ cup of ketchup over it.
- Bake for 50 minutes or until 165°F is detected on a meat thermometer.
- Let cool for five minutes, then serve.

Quinoa Summer Squash Salad

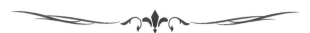

Ingredients
Serves 4

- 1/2 cup of well-rinsed and drained quinoa
- 1 cup chicken or veggie broth
- 2 medium-sized sliced zucchini
- Diced 2 medium yellow squash
- 1/2 tsp salt
- 1/2 teaspoon of black pepper, ground
- 1/2 teaspoon of sage, ground

Steps

- Turn the oven on to 375°F. Position parchment paper on a baking pan.
- Combine the broth and quinoa in a medium saucepan and heat. After stirring to blend, let it boil. After one minute of boiling, cover and turn down the heat. Simmer for 20 minutes, or until the quinoa is tender.

- In a medium bowl, stir zucchini and yellow squash with sage, salt, and pepper while quinoa cooks. Arrange the mixture evenly on the baking sheet and bake for 20 minutes, or until the veggies are tender and caramelized. Take out of the oven and combine with quinoa.
- Serve right away.

Sun-Dried Tomato, Kale, and Bean Salad

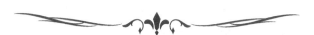

Ingredients
Serves 2

- 2-cups finely chopped kale
- 1 tsp lime juice
- 1 tsp lemon juice
- 1/2 cup washed and drained canned black beans
- 1/2 cup washed and drained canned white beans
- 1/2 cup washed and drained canned kidney beans
- 1/4 cup celery, chopped
- 1/4 tsp salt
- 1/4 teaspoon of black pepper, ground

Steps

- Put the kale in a medium-sized bowl and squeeze in some lemon and lime juice. Massage kale for one to two minutes, or until it begins to soften.

- After adding the last ingredients, toss to coat. For thirty minutes, refrigerate. Present chill.

Salmon Salad Sandwich

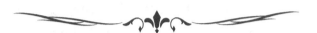

Ingredients
Serves 2

- 1 6-ounce can of wild Alaskan salmon
- 2 tsp finely chopped red onion
- 2 tsp lemon juice
- 1 tsp of vinegar made from apple cider
- 1/4 teaspoon of black pepper, ground
- 4 slices of sprout-grain bread
- 2 tsp of hummus
- 4 tomato slices
- 4 romaine lettuce leaves

Steps
- Combine the salmon, onion, vinegar, lemon juice, and pepper in a small bowl. Put aside.
- After toasting each slice of bread, spread / tbsp of hummus on it.
- Place two tomato slices, two lettuce leaves, and half of the salmon mixture on top of two bread slices. Place the remaining bread on top. Serve right away

Curried Red Lentil Soup

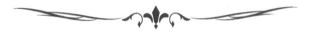

Ingredients
Serves 6

- 1 tablespoon of water.
- 1 big yellow onion, chopped and peeled
- 2 minced garlic cloves
- 1 tablespoon finely chopped fresh ginger
- 1 medium-sized jalapeño jalapeno, seeded, chopped
- 1 tablespoon of curry powder.
- 1 1/2 tablespoons ground cumin.
- 1/2 teaspoon of turmeric powder
- 1 tsp finely ground cinnamon
- Rinse and drain 1 and a half cups of dry red lentils
- 8 cups of chicken broth.
- 1/2 tbsp dried parsley
- 2 tsp lemon juice
- 1 tsp salt
- 1/2 teaspoon of black pepper, ground
- 2 tsp freshly chopped parsley

Steps
- In a large stockpot, heat the water over medium heat. Add the onion and garlic, and sauté for three to four minutes, or until transparent.
- Add the ginger, jalapeño, curry, cumin, turmeric, and cinnamon and simmer for approximately three minutes, or until aromatic.
- Bring the broth to a boil after adding the lentils. Turn down the heat to low and mix in the lemon

- juice, salt, pepper, and dry parsley. Let the lentils cook for 45 to 60 minutes, or until they are tender.
- Add fresh parsley as a garnish.

Chicken and Vegetable Soup

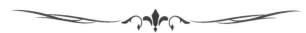

Ingredients
Serves 2

- 2 tsp water
- 8 ounces of cubed, skinless, boneless chicken breasts
- 1 little zucchini, chopped
- 2 medium-sized carrots, sliced and peeled
- 1 medium shallot, peeled, diced
- 2 Roma tomatoes, medium, chopped
- 1 ½ cups baby spinach
- 1 14-oz can of chicken broth
- 2 tablespoons of brown rice, raw
- 1/2 teaspoon of Italian seasoning.
- 1/4 tsp. dry thyme
- 1/4 tsp salt
- 1/4 teaspoon of black pepper, ground

Steps

- Add the cubed chicken to a medium skillet filled with heated water over medium heat. Simmer for 7-8 minutes, or until browned and no longer pink. Using a slotted spoon, remove from the pan.
- Cook the zucchini, carrots, and

- shallot in the pan over medium heat for about 4 minutes, or until they are tender. Add tomatoes and simmer for about 2 minutes, or until barely heated through.
- Place the chicken and vegetable mixture in a large stockpot or saucepan, then top with the other ingredients.
- Over high heat, bring to a boil; after that, lower the heat to a simmer for 20 minutes.

Chicken and Apple Salad

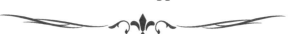

Ingredients
Serves 4

- 1 (12.5-ounce) can of shredded chicken breast.
- 1 medium-sized Granny Smith apple, peeled and cut
- 1 chopped celery stalk
- 2 tsp finely chopped white onion
- 3 tablespoons of chopped sun-dried tomatoes.
- 1 tsp lemon juice
- 1 teaspoon of apple cider vinegar.
- 1/4 tsp seasoned salt
- 1/4 teaspoon of black pepper, ground
- 4 cups of mixed greens

Steps

- In a medium bowl, stir together all ingredients except mixed greens

- until well incorporated. Place on top of mixed greens.

Chapter 4

Dinner Recipes

Shrimp Skewers with Mango Salsa

Ingredients
Serves 2

- 1 small, peeled and diced mango
- 1 sliced green onion
- 3 tsp finely chopped red onion
- 2 tablespoons of finely chopped cilantro
- 1 little jalapeño jalapeno, chopped and seeded
- Juice of 1 large lime plus 2 tablespoons
- 1/8 teaspoon plus ½ teaspoon of salt
- 2 tablespoons of smoked paprika.
- 1½ teaspoon of cumin powder
- 1 tsp finely chopped garlic
- 1/2 teaspoon of black pepper, ground
- 1 pound of raw big shrimp, peeled and deveined.

Steps
- In a big bowl, combine mango, green onion, red onion, cilantro,

jalapeño, lime juice, and / teaspoon salt. For at least half an hour, cover and let it cool.
- As the salsa cools, heat up the grill. In a shallow baking dish, combine paprika, cumin, garlic, remaining salt, pepper, and 2 tablespoons lime juice. Evenly divide the shrimp among the skewers to form kebabs. Put the shrimp kebabs in the marinade and refrigerate for half an hour.
- Shrimp kebabs should be cooked for a full pink color, 2 to 4 minutes on each side.
- Take off the grill, cover with mango salsa, and serve right away.

Pulled Pork with Sweet Potatoes

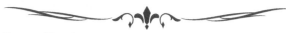

Ingredients
Serves 4

- 1 tsp of chili powder
- 1 tsp ground cumin
- 1 1/2 tsp paprika that has been smoked
- 1 tsp finely ground black pepper

- 1 tsp salt
- 1/2 tspn dry oregano
- 1/4 teaspoon of optional cayenne
- 1-pound pork tenderloin
- 1/4 cup of water
- 2 medium white onions, sliced into rings after peeling.
- 2 medium-sized Gala apples, cored, peeled, and sliced
- 2 medium-sized sweet potatoes, diced and peeling

Steps

- Combine the chili powder, cumin, paprika, pepper, salt, oregano, and cayenne in a small bowl. Make careful to coat the entire pork loin with the spice mixture, getting into all of the nooks and crannies. Refrigerate the pork loin overnight after wrapping it in plastic wrap.
- Before adding water to the slow cooker, lay the onions down in a single layer. Arrange the pork on top of the onions, followed by the apples and sweet potatoes.
- Put the slow cooker on low and cook for 6 hours. Toss the pork with the apple-potato mixture after shredding it with a fork.

Slow Cooker Cilantro Lime Chicken

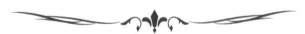

Ingredients
Serves 4

- 1 tablespoon of chili powder.
- 1/4 tsp powdered garlic
- 1/4 teaspoon powdered onion
- 1/4 tspn dry oregano
- 1/2 tsp paprika
- 1 tsp ground cumin
- 1 tsp salt
- 1 tsp finely ground black pepper
- 4 ounces of boneless, skinless chicken breasts
- 1 tiny white onion, chopped and peeled
- 2 minced garlic cloves
- 1 (15.5 ounce) can of black beans, drained and rinsed
- 2 medium-sized limes
- 1 (16-ounce) jar of salsa with no sugar added
- 1½ cups finely chopped cilantro

Steps

- Combine spices in a sizable plastic bag. Coat the chicken breasts by shaking them in a plastic bag.
- Arrange the beans, onion, and garlic along the bottom of a slow cooker. Squeeze lime juice over the beans and place chicken breasts on top. Top with salsa.
- Continue cooking on simmer for 6–8 hours or until the chicken is tender and moist. Before serving, sprinkle some cilantro on top.

Seared Scallop Salad

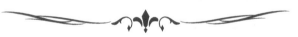

Ingredients
Serves 4

- 1 tsp lemon pepper
- 1 tsp salt
- 2 tablespoons ground black pepper, divided
- 20 huge scallops from the sea
- 8 cups mixed greens.
- 1 cup of grape tomatoes, chopped
- 1/4 cup finely diced red onion
- 1 medium-sized cucumber, cut into slices
- 1/3 cup of mustard
- 1/4 cup of unrefined apple cider vinegar
- 1 tablespoon of water.
- Grill at a medium-high temperature.

Steps

- In a large bowl, mix together lemon pepper, salt, and 1 teaspoon of pepper. Toss the scallops in the basin to coat.
- Scallops should be cooked through after 2-3 minutes on each side of the grill.
- Combine the cucumber, tomatoes, onions, and greens in a big bowl.
- Mix the mustard, vinegar, water, and the remaining teaspoon of pepper in a different small bowl. Drizzle greens with dressing and toss to coat.
- Add scallops on top. Serve right away.

Spaghetti and Meat Sauce

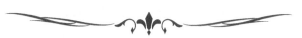

Ingredients
Serves 6

- 1 pound of lean ground beef.
- 1/2 pound of hot, sugar-free Italian pork sausage with the casings removed
- 4 8-ounce cans of tomato sauce (no sugar added)
- 2 6-ounce cans of tomato paste (no sugar added)
- 2 minced garlic cloves
- 2 tsp of Italian seasoning
- 1 tsp salt
- 1/2 teaspoon of black pepper, ground
- 1/2 tsp red pepper flakes
- 6 glasses of water
- 1 pound of brown rice spaghetti.
- 1/2 cup of freshly chopped parsley

Steps

- Cook the Italian sausage and ground beef in a large stockpot over medium-high heat until the meat is no longer pink. Eliminate extra fat.
- Over medium-high heat, add the tomato sauce, tomato paste, garlic, Italian seasoning, salt, black pepper, and red pepper flakes. Boil for one minute, then turn down the heat. Simmer, uncovered, for one hour, stirring now and again.

- Boil water in a separate big pot over high heat. Add the pasta with brown rice. Cook the spaghetti for 6–8 minutes, or until it's the desired doneness, while covered. Place the drained spaghetti into the serving basin.
- Cover the spaghetti with sauce. Add fresh parsley as a garnish.

Chicken Taco Soup

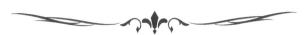

Ingredients
Serves 6

- 1 (15.5 ounce) can of black beans, drained and rinsed
- 1 (15.5 ounce) can of pinto beans, drained and rinsed
- 1 (14.5-ounce) can of fire-roasted chopped tomatoes.
- 1 (12.5 ounce) can of chicken breast in water
- 1 (15-ounce) can of low-fat refried beans.
- 1 (14-ounce) can of chicken broth.
- 1 tablespoon of chili powder.
- 1/4 tsp powdered garlic
- 1/4 teaspoon powdered onion
- 1/4 tspn dry oregano
- 1/2 tsp paprika
- 1 tsp ground cumin
- 1 tsp salt
- 1 tsp finely ground black pepper
- 1 (4-ounce) can of green chiles.

Steps
- Put all ingredients into a slow cooker and stir. Stir until the spices are dissolved.
- Cook for three hours on low heat.

Slow Cooker Adobo Chicken

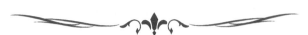

Ingredients
Serves 8

- 1 small sweet onion, peeled and coarsely chopped.
- 1/4 cup of coconut aminos
- 1/4 cup vinegar from red wine
- 1 tsp finely chopped ginger
- 6 smashed garlic cloves
- 1 tsp full black peppercorns
- 2 bay leaves
- 1 whole chicken (4 pounds)

Steps
- Mix the onion, vinegar, coconut aminos, garlic, ginger, peppercorns, and bay leaves in a small bowl.
- Place chicken in slow cooker and cover with mixture. Cook for 6–8 hours on low, or until chicken is well cooked.

Cilantro Lime Chickpea Salad

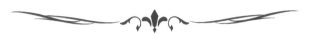

Ingredients
Serves 2

Ingredients
Serves 2

- 1 smashed garlic clove
- 2 tsp hot mustard
- Juice of 1 medium lime
- 1/2 tsp salt
- 1/2 teaspoon of black pepper, ground
- 1 canned (15.5 ounces), washed and drained chickpeas
- 1 (15.5 ounce) can of cannellini beans, drained and rinsed
- 2 cups of finely chopped spinach
- ½ cup finely chopped cilantro
- 1/4 cup finely diced white onion

Steps

- In a small bowl, add the garlic, mustard, lime juice, salt, and pepper, and combine well.
- Chickpeas, cannellini beans, spinach, cilantro, and onion should all be combined in a big bowl.
- Toss to coat after adding the mustard and lime mixture to the chickpea mixture. Chill for thirty to sixty minutes. Present cold.

Sloppy Joes

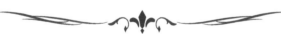

Ingredients
Serves 8

- 2 tablespoons of chicken broth.
- 1 medium-sized yellow onion, sliced and skinned

- 2 minced garlic cloves
- 1 small red bell pepper, chopped and seeded
- 2 pounds of lean ground beef.
- 2 (14.5 ounce) cans of chopped tomatoes
- 1 6-oz can of tomato paste
- 1 cup of sliced mushrooms.
- 2 tsp of coconut aminos
- 2 tsp of chili powder
- 1/2 tsp salt
- 1/2 teaspoon of black pepper, ground

Steps

- In a large skillet, heat the broth over medium-high heat. Add the onion and garlic, and sauté for 4-5 minutes, or until transparent. When the pepper is cooked, add the red pepper and simmer for an additional five minutes. Add the meat and simmer for 6-7 minutes, or until it is no longer pink.
- Place the combination of beef in a slow cooker. After adding the other ingredients, simmer for 4-6 hours on low.

Garlic Pork Roast

Ingredients
Serves 4

- 1 (2-pound) boneless pork shoulder
- 2 tsp salt

- 2 tsp finely ground black pepper
- 5 garlic cloves, cut thinly
- 1 medium-sized yellow onion, sliced and skinned
- 2 medium-sized carrots, sliced and peeled
- 2 celery stalks, diced
- 1 1/2 cup chicken broth.

Steps

- Season the rib roast with salt and pepper. Using a paring knife, make small slits in the pork shoulder. Place a piece of garlic inside each slice.
- Place the pork roast in a slow cooker with celery, carrots, and onion on top. Cover with broth.
- Simmer the pork for 6 hours on low, or until it readily shreds with a fork.

Pumpkin and Sweet Potato Chili

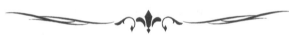

Ingredients
Serves 6

- 1 tsp salt
- 2 tsp of chili powder
- 2 tsp ground cumin
- 1 tsp of dehydrated oregano
- 1/2 tsp ground cinnamon
- 1 tsp powdered unsweetened cocoa
- 1/4 teaspoon of allspice powder
- 2 tsp chicken broth
- 1 tiny white onion, peeled and

- chopped finely
- 2 minced garlic cloves
- 1 pound of lean ground beef.
- 2 medium-sized sweet potatoes, chopped and skinned
- 1 (15-ounce) can of pumpkin puree
- 1 (15.5-ounce) can of fire-roasted diced tomatoes
- 2 cups of beef broth.
- 1/4 cup chopped cilantro
- In a small bowl, combine spices. Put aside.

Steps

- In a large stockpot, warm the broth over medium heat. Add the onion and garlic, and simmer for about 5 minutes, or until transparent. Add the meat and simmer for 6-7 minutes, or until it is no longer pink.
- Stir the spice mixture into the steak until it is well combined.
- Stir to mix the remaining ingredients, excluding the cilantro. Simmer for one hour.
- Garnish with cilantro and serve.

Grilled Flank Steak

Ingredients
Serves 4

- 2 minced garlic cloves
- 1/4 cup of balsamic vinod
- 1/4 cup of coconut aminos

- 2 tsp hot brown mustard
- 2 tsp of rosemary, dried
- 1 tsp of dried thyme
- 1 tsp salt
- 1/2 teaspoon of black pepper, ground
- 1 flank steak weighing 1 pound

Steps

- Combine the garlic, vinegar, coconut aminos, mustard, thyme, rosemary, and salt and pepper in a big mixing basin.
- Place flank steak in a big plastic bag that is sealed. After covering the steak with marinade, seal the bag and press out any extra air. Refrigerate for one hour to marinate.
- Place the steak on the grill grate and preheat it to medium-high heat.
- Cook, coating the steak with marinade, for 6 to 8 minutes on each side, or until desired doneness is reached.
- Steak should be taken off the fire and left for five minutes before slicing.

Slow Cooker Lemon Garlic Chicken

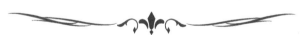

Ingredients
Serves 6

- 2 tsp of dry oregano
- 2 tsp dried parsley

- 1 tsp of seasoned salt
- 1 tsp finely ground black pepper
- 6 (4 ounce) boneless, skinless chicken breasts
- 1/4 cup poultry stock
- 1/4 cup of lemon juice
- 2 minced garlic cloves

Steps

- Put the parsley, oregano, salt, and pepper in a plastic gallon bag. After adding the chicken breasts to the bag, shake to coat.
- Put the chicken breasts in the slow cooker's bottom. Stir in garlic, lemon juice, and broth.
- Simmer the chicken for six hours on low heat, or until it easily flakes with a fork.

Roasted Butternut Squash and Apple Soup

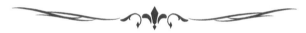

Ingredients
Serves 8

- 1 tsp chicken broth
- 1 medium-sized yellow onion, sliced and skinned
- 8 cups of diced butternut squash.
- 2 medium Granny Smith apples, peeled, cored, and diced
- ½ chopped and seeded medium red bell pepper
- 3 sliced garlic cloves
- 8 cups of vegetable or chicken stock

- 2 tsp salt

Steps
- Heat the chicken stock in a large stockpot over medium-high heat.
- Add the onion and simmer for about 5 minutes, or until transparent. Add the bell pepper, apples, squash, garlic, broth, and salt.
- After bringing to a boil, lower the heat to a simmer for 25 to 30 minutes, or until the squash is soft.
- To purée the ingredients, transfer them to a blender or use an immersion blender.
- Warm up and serve.

Fish Tacos with Pineapple Salsa

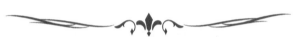

Ingredients
Serves 2

- 1 cup of chopped pineapple.
- 1/4 cup finely chopped red onion
- 1/4 cup finely chopped cilantro and 2 teaspoons added as a garnish
- 1 little jalapeño jalapeno, chopped and seeded
- 1/8 teaspoon plus 1/2 teaspoon salt.
- Juice of 1 medium lime
- 1/2 teaspoon powdered onion
- ½ a teaspoon of powdered garlic
- 1/2 tsp paprika
- 1/2 teaspoon of black pepper, ground

- 2 (6-ounce) haddock fillets.
- 4 (6-") tortillas with sprouted grains

Steps
- In a small bowl, mix together pineapple, red onion, / cilantro, jalapeño, / teaspoon salt, and lime juice. After tossing to mix, chill for an hour.
- With the oven on broil, place an oven rack six inches from the heat source.
- In a small bowl, combine the onion powder, garlic powder, paprika, / teaspoon salt, and pepper.
- Haddock fillets should be placed flat on a foil-lined baking pan. Apply a little coating of the spice blend.
- When the salmon flakes easily with a fork, boil for six minutes.
- Place three ounces of fish and a teaspoon of pineapple salsa on top of each tortilla. If desired, garnish with the remaining cilantro.

Pork Chops with Fresh Applesauce

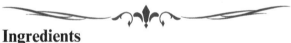

Ingredients
Serves 4

- 1/2 tspn dried thyme
- 1/2 tsp salt
- 1/2 teaspoon of black pepper, ground
- 4 (4 ounce) pork chops, trimmed of fat

- 2 tsp chicken broth
- 4 medium apples, peeled, cored, and diced
- 1 tsp finely ground cinnamon
- 1/8 teaspoon of powdered nutmeg
- 3/4 cup of water
- 2 lemon slices

Steps

- Mix pepper, salt, and thyme in a small basin. Dredge the mixture onto the pork chops.
- Place the broth in a medium-sized skillet and heat it over medium heat.
- When the pork chops are browned and the inside is no longer pink, add them and cook for 5 to 6 minutes on each side. Cover with foil and set aside to rest so it stays heated.
- In a medium-sized saucepan, combine apples, water, nutmeg, cinnamon, and lemon. Over high heat, bring to a boil, then cover and turn down the heat. Stirring often, simmer the apples for 20 minutes or until they are very tender. Take off the heat and put in the food processor. Pulse until smooth or until desired consistency is reached for the applesauce.
- Top with applesauce-topped pork chops. Warm up and serve.

Chicken Sausage with Brown Rice Pasta

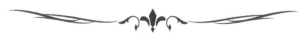

Ingredients
Serves 6

- 6 glasses of water
- 1 (16-ounce) container of brown rice pasta (any flavor).
- 1 12-oz package of sugar-free chicken sausage, cut into quarter-inch-thick coins
- 2 cups of finely chopped spinach
- 1/ cup of roasted red peppers, diced

Steps

- In a large stockpot set over medium-high heat, bring the water to a boil. Cook pasta for 6 to 8 minutes, or until desired consistency is reached, in boiling water. After draining, set away.
- Over medium heat, preheat a medium skillet. Sausage should be cooked in a skillet until browned. Add peppers and spinach to the pan. Cook the spinach for a further three minutes, or until it wilts.
- Cover pasta with sausage mixture.

Vegetable Rice Soup

Ingredients
Serves 4

- 2 tablespoons of water.
- 1 medium-sized yellow onion, sliced and skinned
- 2 minced garlic cloves

- 2 celery stalks, diced
- 2 medium-sized carrots, sliced and peeled
- 1 cup of sliced mushrooms.
- 1 cup of parsnips, diced
- 1 medium-sized, chopped and seeded vine-ripened tomato
- 6 cups of vegetable stock
- 1/2 tsp dried parsley
- 1/4 tsp. dry thyme
- 1/2 tsp salt
- 1/2 teaspoon of black pepper, ground
- 1/4 cup of raw brown rice

Steps

- Heat the water in a large stockpot over medium heat. Cook the onion, garlic, celery, and carrots for five to six minutes, or until they are tender.
- Over high heat, add the other ingredients (excluding rice) and bring to a boil. After five minutes of boiling, turn the heat down to medium.
- After adding the raw rice, simmer the soup for 45 to 60 minutes.
- Warm up and serve.

Tomato Basil Chicken Linguini

Ingredients
Serves 4

- 6 glasses plus 2 tsp water
- Luigi with 8 ounces of brown rice

- 1/2 cup finely chopped white onion
- 2 minced garlic cloves
- 2 cups of freshly chopped tomatoes
- 1/4 cup of freshly chopped basil
- 1/2 tsp salt
- 1/4 teaspoon of black pepper, ground
- 1/2 tsp spicy sauce
- 4 (4-ounce) diced, skinless, boneless chicken breasts

Steps

- In a large pot over medium-high heat, bring 6 cups water to a boil and add the brown rice linguini. Cook for 6 to 8 minutes, or until pasta reaches desired consistency. After draining, set away.
- In a medium skillet, heat 2 tablespoons of water over medium-high heat. Add the onion and garlic, and simmer for about 5 minutes, or until transparent. After three minutes, stir in the tomatoes.
- After adding the remaining ingredients, simmer for about 8 minutes, or until the chicken is no longer pink.
- After adding the chicken mixture to the spaghetti, toss to blend. Serve right away.

Spicy Garlic Chicken

Ingredients
Serves 4

- 1/2 tsp salt
- 1/4 teaspoon of black pepper, ground
- 1/4 teaspoon powdered onion
- 1/4 tsp powdered garlic
- 1/4 teaspoon of paprika, smoked
- 1/8 teaspoon of cayenne
- 1/2 teaspoon of dried parsley
- 4 (4-ounce) boneless, skinless chicken breasts.
- 1/2 fresh medium lime.
- Turn the oven on to 350°F.

Steps

- In a plastic gallon-sized bag, mix together salt, pepper, onion powder, garlic powder, paprika, cayenne, and parsley. To blend, give it a shake.
- To coat the chicken, place it in the bag and shake it.
- After the chicken is thoroughly cooked and its fluids flow clear, place it in a baking dish and bake for 30 minutes. When ready to serve, remove from oven and squeeze lime over chicken breasts.

Chapter 5

Snacks and Sides

Smashed Sweet Potatoes

Ingredients
Serves 4

- 2 big sweet potatoes, split lengthwise in half
- 1/2 tsp salt
- 1/2 tsp ground cinnamon
- 1/4 teaspoon of ground nutmeg (raw)

Steps
- Turn the oven on to 400°F. On a baking sheet, arrange the sweet potatoes cut-side down.
- Bake potatoes for 25 minutes, or until they are tender.
- After taking the potatoes out of the oven, place them in a medium-sized basin.
- Using a potato masher, mash sweet potatoes in their skin.
- Top with nutmeg, cinnamon, and salt, then mash one more.
- Warm up and serve.

Roasted Beets

Ingredients
Serves 4

- 4 large beets, chopped into cubes after peeling
- 1 tsp of dehydrated rosemary
- 1/4 tsp sea salt

Steps
- Turn the oven on to 425°F. Use parchment paper to line a baking sheet.
- Spread out the beets in a single layer on the baking pan and season with sea salt and rosemary.
- Roast until beets are soft, about 15 minutes.

Quinoa Tabbouleh

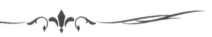

Ingredients
Serves 6

- 1 cup quinoa, rinsed and drained.
- 3 tablespoons lemon juice

- 1 ½ cups water
- 1/2 teaspoon salt
- 1 tsp lime juice
- 1 minced garlic clove
- 2 tsp finely chopped red onion
- 1/2 teaspoon of black pepper, ground
- 2 medium-sized chopped Persian cucumbers
- 1 pint of cherry tomatoes, cut in fourths
- ½ cup finely chopped parsley

Steps

- In a medium saucepan, combine quinoa, water, and salt; cook over medium-high heat. After bringing to a boil, lower the heat to low and cover. Simmer for 10 to 15 minutes, or until water is absorbed and quinoa is soft. Take off the heat and leave covered for a further five minutes. Using a fork, fluff.
- In a large bowl, combine remaining ingredients and stir to combine.
- Add quinoa and toss to coat. Chill for a minimum of one hour prior to serving.

Baked Grapefruit

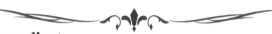

Ingredients
Serves 2

- 1 big pink grapefruit, split in half
- 1½ teaspoon of cinnamon powder
- 1/2 tsp finely chopped ginger

- 1 tsp finely chopped stevia

Steps

- Turn the oven on to 375°F.
- Arrange the grapefruit on the baking sheet, cut side up. Add a quarter of a teaspoon each of cinnamon, ginger, and stevia to each half.
- Bake for fifteen minutes. Warm up and serve.

Red Beans and Rice

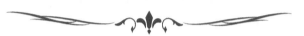

Ingredients
Serves 4

- 2 tsp chicken broth
- 1 little onion, chopped and peeled
- 2 celery stalks, chopped
- 1 tsp salt
- 1/2 teaspoon of black pepper, ground
- 1/8 teaspoon of cayenne
- 2 tablespoons of chopped fresh parsley.
- 1/2 teaspoon dried thyme.
- 1 15.5-oz can of washed and drained red kidney beans
- 2 cups of brown rice, cooked

Steps

- In a medium skillet, heat the broth over medium heat. Add the onion and celery and simmer for about 5 minutes, or until softened.

- After adding the spices and beans, simmer for five minutes. Add rice and stir.
- Warm up and serve.

Balsamic-Glazed Carrots

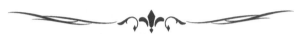

Ingredients
Serves 4

- 3 cups of carrots
- 2 teaspoons of balsamic vinegar.
- 1/4 teaspoon ground black pepper
- 1/2 teaspoon salt
- 1/2 tsp dried parsley

Steps
- Turn the oven on to 400°F. Cover a baking sheet with parchment paper.
- In a big bowl, combine carrots, vinegar, salt, and pepper. Evenly distribute the carrots on the baking pan.
- Carrots should bake for 30 to 40 minutes to get the proper consistency.
- Take out of the oven and add a sprinkle of parsley.

"Creamed" Spinach

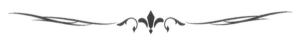

Ingredients
Serves 6

- 2 pounds of raw spinach
- 1/2 cup chicken broth

- 2 minced garlic cloves
- 1 chopped yellow onion
- 1/2 teaspoon salt.
- Juice of 1 big lemon

Steps
- In a double boiler, steam spinach for three minutes, or until it is totally wilted. After letting cool, remove any extra moisture by squeezing.
- In a medium skillet over medium heat, add 1 tablespoon stock and sauté the onion and garlic until tender, about 5 minutes.
- Combine the cooked spinach, onion, and garlic with the remaining broth, salt, and lemon juice in a food processor. Process till everything is smooth.

Spicy Baked Tortilla Chips

Ingredients
Serves 6

- 1 (12-ounce) container of brown rice tortillas
- 2 tsp freshly squeezed lime juice
- 1 tsp ground cumin
- 1/2 tsp chili powder

Steps
- Turn the oven on to 350°F.
- Each tortilla should yield eight triangles, which should be arranged

- in a single layer on a baking sheet. After adding a lime juice drizzle, top with chili powder and cumin.
- Bake until chips are crispy, about 15 minutes.

Black Bean Dip

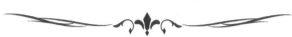

Ingredients
Serves 4

- 1 (15.5 ounce) can of black beans, drained and rinsed
- 1/2 cup finely sliced yellow onion
- 2 minced garlic cloves
- 1 tsp ground cumin
- 1/2 teaspoon chili powder.
- 1/2 tsp salt
- 2 TEASOPS of tomato paste
- 1 tablespoon of fresh lime juice.
- 1 tablespoon of chopped green chilies.
- 2 chopped green onions
- 1/4 cup of finely chopped cilantro

Steps
- Blend beans, tomato paste, onion, garlic, cumin, chili powder, salt, and lime juice in a food processor until smooth.
- Add the green chilies and garnish with cilantro and green onions.

Simple Quinoa

Ingredients

Serves 4

- 1 cup quinoa, rinsed and drained.
- 1/2 teaspoon garlic salt
- 2 cups vegetable broth
- 1 tsp freshly squeezed lemon juice

Steps
- Place the quinoa and stock in a medium saucepan and bring to a high boil. After bringing to a boil, lower the heat to a simmer and cover.
- Simmer for 20 minutes, or until the quinoa is fluffy and soft.
- Using a fork, fluff the quinoa and mix in the lemon juice and garlic salt.
- Warm up and serve.

Fruit Salad

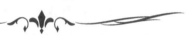

Ingredients
Serves 4

- 1 cup of cantaloupe, diced
- 1 cup of chopped honeydew.
- 1 cup diced pineapple.
- 1 cup of hulled and halved strawberries
- 1 tsp finely ground cinnamon
- 1/2 tsp finely chopped stevia

Steps
- In a large bowl, combine all ingredients and toss to coat. Let it cool for at least half an hour before

serving.

Turnip Fries

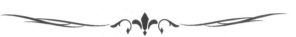

Ingredients
Serves 2

- 4 little turnips, peeled and sliced into sticks measuring 2"
- 1/4 tsp salt
- 1/4 tsp powdered black pepper
- 1/4 teaspoon of hot sauce

Steps
- Turn the oven on to 425°F.
- Arrange the turnip sticks on a baking sheet coated with foil.
- Toss turnips with a little salt, pepper, and chili powder.
- Disperse into a solitary layer. Fries should be baked for 15 minutes, then flipped over and baked for an additional 15 minutes. Warm up and serve.

Pumpkin Pie Apple Slices

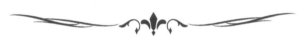

Ingredients
Serves 2

- 2 teaspoons of pumpkin pie spice.
- 1 tsp finely chopped stevia
- 2 medium Granny Smith apples, cored and thinly sliced
- 2 tsp lemon juice
- 2 tsp water

Steps
- Put stevia and pumpkin pie spice in a plastic gallon bag. After soaking for half an hour in a medium-sized bowl with lemon juice, place the apple slices in a plastic bag with pumpkin pie spice and shake to coat the apples.
- Add the coated apples to a medium saucepan filled with water set over medium heat. Cook for five minutes, or until apples are soft and toasty. Warm up and serve.

Roast Beef and Pickle Wraps

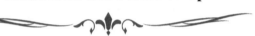

Ingredients
Serves 2

- 4 thinly sliced (4 ounces) of nitrate-free roast meat
- 4 spears of medium-dill pickles

Steps
- Halve each pickle spear and each slice of roast meat.
- Use a toothpick to secure each pickle spear after rolling it in roast meat.
- Serve right away.

Summer Squash Bake

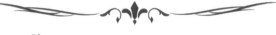

Ingredients
Serves 4

- 2 medium zucchini chopped into 1/4" rounds.
- Cut 2 medium yellow summer squashes into ¼ -inch circles.
- 2 tsp of Italian seasoning
- 2 minced garlic cloves
- 1/2 tsp salt
- 1/2 teaspoon of black pepper, ground

Steps

- Turn the oven on to 375°F.
- In a medium bowl, toss the sliced squash and zucchini with the spice, garlic, salt, and pepper.
- Transfer to a baking dish, then bake for ten minutes. After flipping, heat for a further five minutes, or until the food is tender.

Mashed Parsnips

Ingredients
Serves 6

- 4 pounds of quartered and peeled parsnips
- 1 cup chicken broth
- 1/2 teaspoon ground black pepper
- 1 teaspoon salt
- 2 tablespoons of chives

Steps

- Fill a large stockpot halfway full of water and add parsnips. Bring to a boil over high heat, then lower the heat to a simmer for about 20

- minutes, or until the parsnips are tender. Empty.
- Process the parsnips, broth, salt, and pepper in a food processor until smooth.
- Add the chives and stir. Serve right away.

Garlic Zucchini Noodles

Ingredients
Serves 4

- 6 medium zucchini, thinly sliced or spiralized using a spiralizer
- 1 tsp salt
- 1 tbsp chicken broth
- 2 minced garlic cloves

Steps

- After adding salt, let the zucchini "sweat" for thirty minutes. Chill the zucchini with a paper towel.
- In a medium skillet, heat the broth over medium heat. Add the garlic and simmer for 3 minutes or until fragrant.
- Cook the zucchini "noodles" for about five minutes, or until they are soft. Take care to avoid overcooking.

Mexican Brown Rice

Ingredients
Serves 4

- 1 cup brown rice.
- 1/2 teaspoon salt
- 1 ½ cups of water
- 1/2 (15.5-ounce) can of fire-roasted diced tomatoes.
- 1½ cups finely chopped cilantro

Steps

- In a medium saucepan, mix rice, water, and salt together. Increase heat to high, bring to a boil, cover, and lower heat to low. Simmer for 20 minutes, or until rice is tender and water is absorbed.
- Take off the heat and use a fork to fluff.
- Stir in tomatoes and cilantro after adding them.

Sausage and Apple Stuffing

Ingredients
Serves 4

- 2 little sweet potatoes, chopped and skinned
- Cut and core 2 medium Granny Smith apples.
- 1 tablespoon of water.
- 1 little yellow onion, chopped and peeled
- 2 chopped celery stalks
- 1/2 pound of Italian sausage without the casings
- 1/2 tsp salt
- 1/2 tsp ground black pepper
- 1/2 teaspoon of sage, ground

Steps

- Turn the oven on to 400°F. Use parchment paper to line a baking sheet.
- Spread the chopped sweet potatoes and apples in a single layer on the baking sheet after tossing them together. After around 30 minutes, roast until soft and beginning to turn golden.
- In a medium skillet, heat the water over medium-high heat. Add the onion and celery, and simmer for about 5 minutes, or until softened.
- Sausage, salt, pepper, and sage should be added. Cook for about 7 minutes, or until sausage is no longer pink.
- After letting the sausage cool for five minutes, add it to the sweet potato and apple mixture and toss to blend.

Quinoa Pilaf

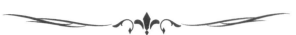

Ingredients
Serves 2

- 3 cups plus 2 tablespoons of chicken broth
- 1 chopped small shallot
- 1/2 cup of white mushrooms, sliced
- 2 medium-sized carrots, sliced and peeled
- 1 and a half cups of rinsed and drained quinoa

- 1 tsp salt
- 1/2 teaspoon of black pepper, ground
- 1/4 cup of freshly chopped parsley

Steps

- In a medium saucepan, warm up two tablespoons of broth over medium heat. Add the shallots and sauté for about 3 minutes, or until softened. Cook the carrots and mushrooms for an additional five minutes, or until they are tender.
- Stir the quinoa and remaining broth together until well incorporated. Over high heat, bring to a boil, then lower the heat to a simmer and cover. Simmer for 20 minutes, or until the quinoa is fluffy and soft.
- Using a fork, fluff the mixture and mix in the parsley, salt, and pepper. Warm up and serve.

MEAL PLANNER

	BREAKFAST	LUNCH	DINNER	SNACKS
MON				
TUES				
WED				
THURS				
FRI				
SAT				
SUN				

MEAL PLANNER

	BREAKFAST	LUNCH	DINNER	SNACKS
MON				
TUES				
WED				
THURS				
FRI				
SAT				
SUN				

MEAL PLANNER

	BREAKFAST	LUNCH	DINNER	SNACKS
MON				
TUES				
WED				
THURS				
FRI				
SAT				
SUN				

MEAL PLANNER

	BREAKFAST	LUNCH	DINNER	SNACKS
MON				
TUES				
WED				
THURS				
FRI				
SAT				
SUN				

MEAL PLANNER

	BREAKFAST	LUNCH	DINNER	SNACKS
MON				
TUES				
WED				
THURS				
FRI				
SAT				
SUN				

MEAL PLANNER

	BREAKFAST	LUNCH	DINNER	SNACKS
MON				
TUES				
WED				
THURS				
FRI				
SAT				
SUN				

MEAL PLANNER

	BREAKFAST	LUNCH	DINNER	SNACKS
MON				
TUES				
WED				
THURS				
FRI				
SAT				
SUN				

MEAL PLANNER

	BREAKFAST	LUNCH	DINNER	SNACKS
MON				
TUES				
WED				
THURS				
FRI				
SAT				
SUN				

MEAL PLANNER

	BREAKFAST	LUNCH	DINNER	SNACKS
MON				
TUES				
WED				
THURS				
FRI				
SAT				
SUN				

MEAL PLANNER

	BREAKFAST	LUNCH	DINNER	SNACKS
MON				
TUES				
WED				
THURS				
FRI				
SAT				
SUN				

MEAL PLANNER

	BREAKFAST	LUNCH	DINNER	SNACKS
MON				
TUES				
WED				
THURS				
FRI				
SAT				
SUN				

MEAL PLANNER

	BREAKFAST	LUNCH	DINNER	SNACKS
MON				
TUES				
WED				
THURS				
FRI				
SAT				
SUN				

Thank You

Thank you for choosing "THE GOOD ENERGY COOKBOOK." It has been a labor of love, and I am deeply grateful that you've taken the time to explore these recipes and ideas with me. My hope is that this book brings you as much joy, health, and energy as it has brought to my own life.

Creating this book has been a journey, and I couldn't have done it without the support of my friends, family, and everyone who has inspired me along the way. A special thank you to those who provided feedback, encouragement, and endless taste-testing during the creation process.

If you found "THE GOOD ENERGY COOKBOOK" helpful, I would be incredibly grateful if you could take a moment to leave an honest review on Amazon. Your feedback not only helps others discover the book but also supports my ongoing work in bringing more healthy, energy-boosting recipes to life.

Thank you for being a part of this journey. Wishing you good health, happiness, and boundless energy!

With gratitude,
Jacqueline L. Payne

Made in United States
Troutdale, OR
09/03/2024

22549226R00040